This new edition of a Victorian waterways classic,
describing a boating trip from the Thames at
Weybridge to the South Coast via the Wey and Arun
Canal is
DEDICATED
by the Publisher to members of the Wey and Arun
Canal Trust Ltd, who are striving to reopen the
Lost Route. A proportion of the Publisher's
royalties is being given to the Trust to help them
towards their objective.

ISBN 0 906986 00 1
This book was first published in 1868
by Longmans, Green & Co.
This edition published in 1980.
© Cover design, Foreword and Publisher's
Introduction, Shepperton Swan.

Printed in Great Britain by
Manson Graphic, 12 Frogmore Road, Apsley,
Hemel Hempstead, Hertfordshire
for Shepperton Swan, The Clock House,
Upper Halliford, Shepperton, Middlesex. TW17 8RU.

THE LOG

OF

'THE CAPRICE.'

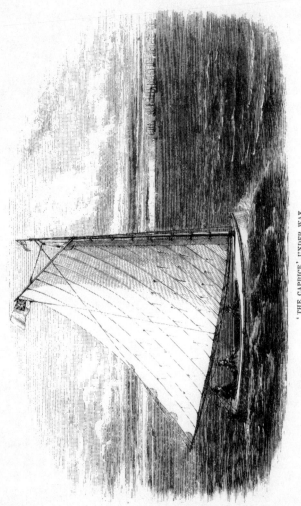

'THE CAPRICE' UNDER WAY.

THE THAMES TO THE SOLENT

BY CANAL AND SEA

OR

THE LOG OF THE UNA BOAT 'CAPRICE.'

BY

J. B. DASHWOOD.

LONDON:

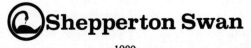
Shepperton Swan

1980

PUBLISHER'S INTRODUCTION TO THIS NEW EDITION

THIS charming waterways travelogue is one of the earliest accounts of pleasure cruising on canals. When it first appeared in 1868 (at a price of 2s6d (12½p), its very unusualness attracted considerable attention, one review in *The Chromolithograph* describing it as "a pleasantly written narrative . . . a novel description of a voyage." Over the century that has elapsed since Mr and Mrs Dashwood made their journey, this book has acquired a reputation as one of the most sought-after canal books of the 1800s. It has not been unknown for avid collectors of waterways literature to pay up to £50 for an original copy.

By republishing *The Thames to the Solent by Canal and Sea,* I am delighted to be able to introduce modern readers to one of my favourite books. If its reappearance does even a little to encourage restoration of the long-closed, much-regretted Wey and Arun Canal, I shall be more than pleased.

A first-rate and copious account of the history of these waterways is contained in *London's Lost Route to the Sea,* by P.A.L. Vine (David & Charles, 1965 and subsequent editions.)

Since Dashwood's day, inland cruising has achieved undreamed-of popularity. He would doubtless marvel at the present scope of the canal boating industry in Britain, an activity where he was one of the very first pioneers.

HUGH McKNIGHT

FOREWORD BY PETER BERESFORD, CHAIRMAN, WEY & ARUN CANAL TRUST LTD.

WHEN the Wey and Arun Canal Trust heard that this book was to be reprinted the reaction was one of great enthusiasm. Very few of the Trust's members have had the opportunity to read this rare classic account, although many *Caprices* reside in people's imaginations (and in more tangible forms!) awaiting the day when it will be possible to emulate Dashwood and again navigate the Wey and Arun Canal for pleasure.

The Wey and Arun Canal was opened throughout in 1816. Trade got off to a slow start, and although the Canal prospered in the 1830s, the coming of the railways caused a rapid decline in the Canal's fortunes, the Wey and Arun Canal closing in 1868, and being legally abandoned in 1871.

The rural situation of the Canal which failed to provide sufficient trade during its working life has probably been responsible for the preservation of its line, which lay as a truly 'forgotten' waterway until the Wey and Arun Canal Society was formed in 1970 to restore the navigable link between the River Wey and the South Coast, this society later becoming the Wey and Arun Canal Trust Ltd. The line of the Canal has remained almost completely intact, the countryside through which it passes being much as Dashwood found it, although the Canal itself has suffered from the effects of a century's vegetation.

If the readers of this book are tempted to seek out the route of the Canal, as we are sure many will be, may we stress the importance of 'explorers' keeping to the public rights of way, as the land through which the Canal passes is privately owned. A guide to walking the Canal is available from the Trust.

Although the Canal itself remains, the locks, bridges, etc. are a different matter. Dashwood found the Canal in disrepair so it is no surprise that many of the structures have vanished completely. The Trust is confident that the Canal will be re-opened, although it is obviously a long-term project. Any account of the Trust's work so far is out of date as soon as it is published, so suffice it to say that by the tenth birthday of our restoration movement we are well on the way to having achieved five bridges restored, rebuilt or built from scratch, two locks brought into a potentially usable condition and several miles of canal bed cleared and returned to water (although keeping the water is as great a problem now as in Dashwood's day!).

The Trust asks for as much support as possible — not only on the weekly working parties or the fund raising activities, but simply by adding another name to the hundreds who have already endorsed our work will the visible support for the Trust be enhanced and the sooner will the latter-day *Caprices* be able to re-live Dashwood's experiences.

October 1979.

PREFACE.

—◦◦—

AMONGST the many works written on sailing, rowing, shooting and fishing upon the Thames, the author has not yet met with an account of a trip from thence to the Solent by canal, which forms the subject of this little book.

This 'voyage' was accomplished in a small Una-rigged boat, which gives the writer the opportunity of offering the results of his experience with regard to the capabilities of these little vessels for river and sea sailing, as well as for fishing and shooting.

As the reader will perceive, the expedition from Weybridge to Portsmouth can be made (wind and weather permitting) in four or five days, so that a fortnight's holiday may, in this way, be agreeably spent.

The following incidents were originally put upon paper merely as memoranda of this pleasant journey, but the writer having received so many assurances from his friends that the subject would be of interest· to the general public, he has ventured to publish them, hoping that they may prove entertaining and useful.

The descriptions (historical and topographical) of the various places of interest on the route have been in a great measure taken from Murray's Handbooks of Surrey and Sussex, as well as from the 'Beauties of England and Wales.'

The last chapter is essentially a nautical one, and has nothing to say to the expedition. It has been written with the sole purpose of giving the writer's experience with regard to Unarigged boats, and contains several suggestions which he trusts may prove of use. As this chapter is written solely for nautical readers, it is hoped the unsophisticated will not find fault with the nautical terms.

J.B. DASHWOOD

CONTENTS.

CHAPTER I.

CHAPTER II.

CHAPTER III.

CONTENTS.

CHAPTER IV.

CHAPTER V.

CHAPTER VI.

CHAPTER VII.

ILLUSTRATIONS.

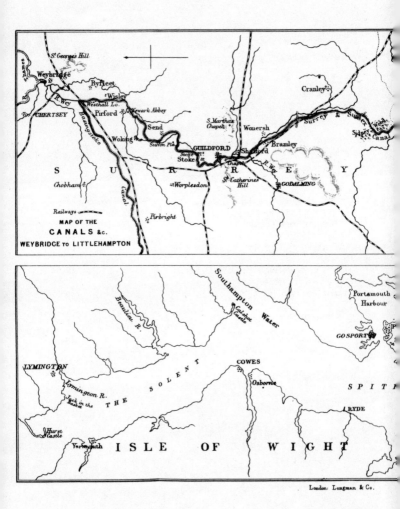

MAP OF THE
CANALS &c.
WEYBRIDGE TO LITTLEHAMPTON

Railways ++++++++

London: Longman & Co.

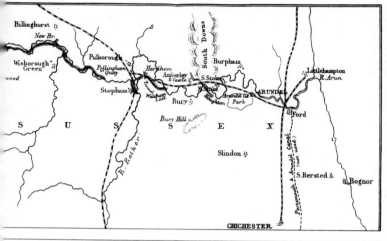

Billinghurst
New Br.
Wisborough
Green
wood
Pulborough
Pollingham Quay
Hardham
Harttham Quay
Amberley
& Castle
South Downs
Burpham
S. Stoke
Stopham
Waldam Lock
W. Stoke
Houghton
Arundel Ct.
Park
ARUNDEL
Littlehampton
R. Arun
Bury
Ford
S U S S E X
R. Rother
Bury Hill
Slindon
Portsmouth & Arundel Canal (not used)
S. Bersted
Bognor
CHICHESTER

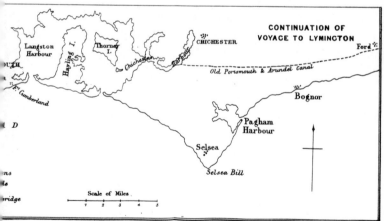

CONTINUATION OF
VOYAGE TO LYMINGTON

Langston
Harbour
Hayling I.
Thorney
I.
Chichester
CHICHESTER
Bosham
Ford
Old Portsmouth & Arundel Canal
OUTH
R. Cumberland
D
Bognor
Pagham
Harbour
Selsea
ns
le
ridge
Selsea Bill

Scale of Miles
1 2 3 4 5

FROM

THE THAMES TO THE SOLENT.

———•◦•———

CHAPTER I.

AT twelve o'clock on the morning of July 8,
1867, the little Una boat 'Caprice' weighed
anchor on her voyage from Weybridge to the
Solent. The day was lovely, and all seemed to
smile success on this adventurous expedition.
Her crew consisted of your humble servant and
his better half, attended by their faithful and
devoted dog Buz, of the true Pomeranian breed.
We had placed all we required for our toilette
in a small portmanteau, and in addition, had
provided ourselves with a portable india-rubber
bath, a ship's compass, a basket jar of four
gallons for water, a small keg to contain a gallon

B

of beer, a luncheon basket fitted with plates, knives, forks, cups, &c. &c, a cooking apparatus, and last, though not least, a complete foul-weather rig of overalls, rugs, umbrellas, &c.

It was necessary, before starting by canal, to unship the mast, which is 20 feet long, and to substitute a short towing mast, seven feet in length, in its place. The sailing mast we lashed to the boom, and stowed all away in such a manner as not to interfere with our comfort nor with the proper working of the helm.

It may perhaps be as well to mention that we attached a small block to the head of the towing mast, through which we passed the towing line (30 yards long) and made it fast to the cleat inside the boat—this we found the best plan, for on starting we could at all times ease it off and prevent a sudden strain, which would have been injurious to the boat.

Several of our friends, in the kindness of their hearts, came down to the river's banks to see us off, and having supplied us with cake and fruit, wished us ' Good speed.'

The oars were out, and we paddled her up to the first lock on the Wey. Here we were called upon to pay a toll of five shillings, which freed us as far as Guildford. Our next care was to provide ourselves with a crowbar, three feet long,

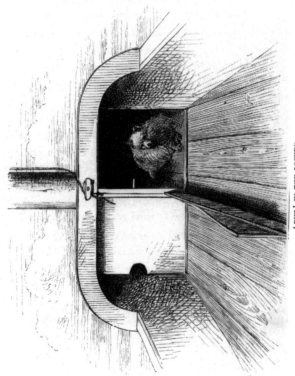

'BUZ' IN THE LOCKER.

for opening the locks (ten in number) between Weybridge and Guildford.

The lock-keeper at Weybridge we found most civil and obliging, and he readily lent us the magic wand which passed us from one end of this part of the canal to the other. Although possessed of this formidable weapon, let me counsel those who are not adepts at its use to beware how they trifle with it, lest perchance they either inflict woeful wounds on their hands, or worse than all, fall headlong into the lock. The hatches of many of these locks are placed, goodness knows why, in the very centre of the gates, and in order to open and shut them, it is necessary to sit astride the gates, place the point of the crowbar in the niches of the hatch, and by violent jerks raise it inch by inch until the flood gates are opened. These hatches are always very stiff and difficult to raise and lower, and as it is necessary to get a good leverage, the crowbar must be worked from the extreme end of the handle, and if, whilst the wrench is made, the point should slip out of the niche into which it is placed, away goes the unfortunate being into the water.*

We fortunately received a lesson in the art of lock opening from a Cambridge friend, who

* See Illustration, p. 16.

kindly voluntered to show us the knack, and thereby put us *au fait* of opening these annoying, though useful obstacles to our journey. He accompanied us through the second lock, and having imparted a warning to me to be careful how I dealt with these infernal machines, I am happy to say I got through our journey without a ducking, though not without some reminiscences of my labours in the shape of cuts and bruizes.

After passing through the first lock, we were met by our groom, George Keene, leading a favorite dark chesnut pony, 14 hands high, whose duty it was to tow the boat until we reached the sea. This little mare had been our companion and constant helper on many a former trip through North Wales and various parts of England; a better bred little animal could not well be found; our only doubt was, would she be quiet enough for the purpose for which she was now intended? But why did we for a moment doubt? nothing could have exceeded the patience and endurance with which she performed her part of the task.

A word or two on the subject of the towing-gear may not here be out of place. There are two or more ways of harnessing a horse for towing—the plan adopted by most of the bar-

gees on the Thames, is to have the traces long
enough to extend two or more feet behind the
horse, so that, when the beast is suddenly halted,
the splinter bar, to which the traces and tow-
ropes are attached, falls to the ground, and in no
way interferes with the animal's hocks. My
objection, however, to this plan is that the horse
is liable to get his legs over the traces whilst
they lie on the ground, which would in nine
cases out of ten, with a spirited animal, occasion
accident. The plan we adopted was to have
the traces just so long as to allow the splinter
bar to rest a little above the hocks, but not short
enough to impede the free action of the pony.
The traces were kept up by means of a kicking
strap passed through the crupper, attached to
the saddle. At first the pony did not much ap-
prove of this new style of harness, but in a
very short time became quite accustomed to it,
and during our journey we found no difficulty
whatever on this score. The collar should be
well padded and fit the horse perfectly, and
the trace farthest away from the boat, whilst
towing, should be let out one hole longer than
the near one, if possible, but in cases where the
towing path is frequently shifted from one side
of the river to the other, the time taken up in
shortening the one trace and letting out the

other would occasion, perhaps, too much delay, but if it can be done—say, whilst the locks are being opened or during any stoppage—it will be found to give a more even strain on the shoulders of the horse, and greater steadiness to the motion of the boat.

The towing line should be made fast to the splinter bar in three places, namely from the centre and two ends ; if this is not attended to, a jerking motion, most disagreeable, will take place ; the bar will in all probability be snapped in half ; and in any case, it will be perpetually swinging in all directions.

I trust that my readers who are already thoroughly acquainted with the knack of tow-ing will pardon these remarks, which I have thought might be of some practical use to the uninitiated.

CHAPTER II.

WEYBRIDGE TO GUILDFORD.

OBSTACLES IN THE WAY—NEWARK PRIORY—PIRFORD LOCK—
SEND—WOKING CHURCH—RUINS OF AN OLD ROYAL PALACE—
SUTTON PLACE—ORIGIN OF LOCKS IN ENGLAND—SAINFOIN
AND TURNIPS FIRST INTRODUCED INTO THIS COUNTRY—STOKE
—ARRIVAL AT GUILDFORD.

BEING now fairly under way, we soon left Weybridge astern, and to our joy found ourselves
entering into a long and beautiful avenue of
high alders. The canal at this point was very
lovely, about 15 feet wide, the trees growing in
the water on either side; the avenue was about
three miles long, with here and there pretty rustic
bridges spanning the stream. The day was hot
and the cool shade most refreshing, the banks
were covered with luxuriant ferns and wild flowers,
and the white and yellow water lilies, floating on
the smooth surface of the water, lent enchant-
ment to the view. A fly-rod skilfully worked
might at this time have had some fine sport, for
the fish were rising in all directions most greedily.

Our object however was to get on, and to introduce our little craft to the saline waters of the
deep.   At the end of this pretty bit of scenery
we emerged upon New Haw lock, a very large
deep lock, requiring considerable force to work;
we happily at this point came up with a barge,
like ourselves ascending the canal : they offered
us their services, which were readily accepted,
and in ten minutes we had mounted about
ten feet higher, and found ourselves in a more
open country of meadow and corn-fields.   On
our left the scene was shut in by the pretty wood-
lands of St. George's Hill and the line of the
Surrey Hills in every form of undulation, wrapped
in a lovely purple haze, which indicated a long
continuance of fine weather ; the foreground was
alive with hay-makers ; and the whole would
have formed a charming subject for the brush
of a Linnell or a Copley Fielding.

On our right we soon came to a pretty place
called Westhall Lodge, standing in the midst of
its farm ; at the time we passed, the inmates were
busily enjoying themselves in the all-enthralling
game of croquet.   So we travelled on slowly and
surely, at a pace of about four miles an hour, in-
cluding the locks, which took us on an average,
single-handed, about 15 minutes each to open,
though a stiff one would take as long as 20
minutes.

One of the greatest hindrances to our rapid progress was the endless number of gates across the towing-path, all of which were swinging five-barred gates. With a steady-going nag, the best and quickest way of getting through them is to have a hunting-crop in hand, with which to swing them open, and to go through at a brisk trot, the man on board the boat being always ready to haul the rope taut, and with a jerk, to clear it of the gate before it shuts-to again.

The country beyond this is not particularly striking; the canal passes by Wisley Common, and on until we reach Newark Lock.

Here, on the right, lie the interesting ruins of Newark Priory, on a site originally named Aldebury, and also called Newsted, and De Novo Loco in the early charters. It was formerly occupied by Augustinian canons, and was founded by Rual de Calva in the days of Richard Cœur de Lion. The Priory was dedicated to the Virgin and St. Thomas of Canterbury, and received at different times extensive grants of land. Its annual revenue at the dissolution, 26 Henry VIII., was 258*l*. 11*s*. 11*d*.; the last prior was Richard Lippiscomb, who enjoyed a pension of 40*l*. per annum. In 1556 the monastery and its possessions were granted to Sir A. Brown, and descended to Lord Montacute, subsequently to Earl Onslow, and are now the property of Lord Lovelace. A footpath leads from the river to the ruins, whose gray walls rise in sharp contrast with the deep bright green of the adjoining meadows. They are of Early English character. The walls are very thick, and composed of flint and hard mortar. The portion which still stands is most probably a part of the Priory church, and it is said that a subterranean passage led under the river to a nunnery in the parish of Ockham.

The surrounding scenery is composed of rivers and rivulets (seven streams run by the Priory, according to Aubrey), 'footbridges and fords, plashy pools and fringed tangled hollows, trees in groups or alone, and cattle dotted over the pastures.'

Adjoining Newark Lock on the left is Newark Mill, and a stone bridge here crosses the river.

Whilst the lock was filling, I took the opportunity of running across the fields a distance of about a hundred yards to inspect the ruins.

The same open scenery, flat pastures, distant woods, with the Surrey hills beyond, continued until we reached Pirford Lock, about two miles from Newark. Here we brought up for a rest, and procured some bread and cheese from a

little inn adjoining the lock. The inn was full
of weary haymakers, who asked me in a plain-
tive voice if it was not *very* hot. I suggested in
reply that some beer might be refreshing, and
ordered it for them. Their joy may be ima-
gined, and I was amply repaid, for they rushed
out, insisting on filling the lock themselves.

After passing through Walsam and Pepper-
court Locks, we arrived at the village of Send.
Here we baited the pony, and ate our luncheon
under the shade of some fine alders growing on
the water's edge, after which we strolled about
to see the place. The village is small, with a
nice inn, where refreshments simple and clean
can be obtained. The church is a large Perpendicular building covered with ivy, but con-
taining nothing of any note. In the church-
yard are some fine elms.

On the opposite side of the river, about a mile
off, is situated the town of Woking, where the
traveller may find good quarters at the White
Hart, and should he be fond of architecture and
the picturesque, let him walk down to the old
church just outside the town. The tower is old
and covered with moss. The chancel is Early
English, but the rest of the church is of more
modern date. Aubrey, on the information of
the sexton, relates that as long as there are any

remains of a corpse besides bones in the church-
yard of Woking, a kind of plant about the
thickness of a bulrush, with a top like the
head of asparagus, grows from it, and shoots up
nearly to the surface of the earth, above which
it never appears; and that when the corpse is
quite consumed, the plant dies away. He adds
that the same observation has been made at
Send, and in other churchyards where the soil
is a light red sand, as at Woking.

A short distance below Woking are still to be
seen the foundations of a palace chiefly of very
fine brick, which was the occasional residence
of Edward IV., Henry VII. and Henry VIII.
At length James I., by letters-patent, granted
the manor to Sir Edward Zouch, from whom it
descended to Lord Onslow. The walls of one
room are still existing, which is said to have
been the guardroom during the residence in
the palace of the Sovereign. It was here that
Wolsey, when Archbishop of York, received the
intimation that he had been elected a Cardinal.
On the hill-top, the remains of a tower capped
by a kind of lantern still exist, which is said to
have been used for the king's guidance when
he came to visit Sir Edward Zouch at night.
Sir Edward Zouch, according to Sir Anthony
Weldon, was one of the ' chief and master fools '
who assisted in the king's pastimes.

It was now time for us to get under weigh
again, and to proceed on our journey. We lost
no time in putting to, and went off at a brisk
trot. We soon came to another lock, called
Triggs Lock, which we passed without much
trouble. As we neared Guildford, the scenery
became much more interesting; we had left the
flat country behind us at Woking, and were
approaching the Surrey hills.

We now entered Sutton Place, a beautiful
park, the property of Captain Salvin; the woods
on either side of the river were rich in foliage,
and so perfectly arranged in groups as to be
quite a *chef d'œuvre* of landscape gardening;
immediately below the woods, the haymakers
were busy at work loading their waggons. The
day was now advancing, and the great heat had
given place to a calm and lovely evening. We
thoroughly enjoyed our journey as we glided
along the banks gay with the water-iris, both
yellow and blue, the pretty little forget-me-nots
in quantities, the large yellow ranunculus, with
no end of other pretty wild flowers, the air
fragrant with the scent of new-mown hay and
the delicious smelling meadow-sweet.

Before we proceed further on our journey, let
us stop and have a look at this interesting old
place. The house stands on high ground above

the river. It was built in 1530 by Sir R. Weston, to whom King Henry VIII. granted the manor. Sir Richard Weston was father of Francis Weston, gentleman of the privy chamber to Henry VIII., who was involved in the fate of Anne Boleyn, and beheaded on Tower Hill. The mansion is in the form of a parallelogram, and built of red brick, furnished with a double sculptured plat-band of terra-cotta running round the top, with coins and window-cases of the same, giving an imposing richness to the exterior. Many of the bricks are marked with the initials R. W., and a tun, with bunches of hops encircled by an ornamental border, in allusion to Sir Richard Weston having been brewer to Henry VIII. Some of the windows in the north and south fronts, with their mullions of terra-cotta beautifully moulded, remain in a perfect state of preservation.

The great hall, which occupies the centre of the edifice, is 50 feet long, 25 feet wide, and 31 feet high, and contains some fine windows, with shields representing the cognisances of Edward IV. (the rose *en soleil*) and of Henry VII. (the crown in a hawthorn bush), besides the various roses of the Tudor sovereigns. The other devices seem later, that of the clown crossing a brook with five goslings tucked under his belt, is probably copied from Withers' ' Emblems,' published in 1635, where 'a fool sent forth to fetch the goslings home' is said to have thrust them under his girdle, and so strangled them, for fear they should be drowned in crossing a river.

> The best good turns that fools can do us
> Prove disadvantages unto us.

is Withers' moral (A. J. Kempe). The south-east front has a long gallery 141 feet in length, 20 feet in width, and 14 feet in height, where Queen Elizabeth was entertained in 1591. Immediately after her departure, a fire broke out in this part of the building, and the whole of the woodwork was entirely consumed. This portion was rebuilt in 1721. Under the gallery, on the ground floor, are four fine rooms, which have never been fitted up for use.

According to Aubrey, Sir Richard Weston, great-grandson of the first grantee, in the year 1645, introduced into this country the first clover-grass, and probably sainfoin and turnips, out of Brabant or Flanders. To Sir Richard Weston we are likewise indebted for our navigation by canal, for he was the first to introduce the system of locks, and he it was who first rendered the Wey navigable; an Act of Parliament for carrying his projects into effect was passed in the year 1651.

We must now resume our journey. After passing Bowers Lock, we soon arrive at Stoke, a suburb of Guildford. Stoke Park lies on the left bank of the river, and is hilly and prettily wooded.

At Stoke Mill we came to our last lock before Guildford: a very deep one it was, and one of the most difficult to work: by this time, however, I had become pretty handy with the crowbar, and we were not long in getting through. The toll-keeper here emerged from the neighbouring flour mill and demanded our way-bill, and to him I gave up, without much reluctance, the ponderous instrument which had helped us so far on our way, with an injunction to send it back by the first opportunity to the lock-keeper at Weybridge.

'The shades of night were falling fast,' and we had two miles more to Guildford, which we accomplished in about half an hour, entering the old town in the twilight of evening. We were somewhat tired with our day's work, and were not sorry to pull up under the old bridge, where we left our boat for the night, in charge of the boatman on the quay. The town was alive with excitement, it being the Foresters' fête, and Volunteers' bands paraded the streets in every direction. Guildford has always a

WORKING THE LOCKS.

great charm for me, but this evening all was so merry and jolly that it quite gladdened our hearts as we made the best of our way to the White Lion, anxious for our dinner, it being then past nine o'clock, and with the intention of remaining there for the night.

CHAPTER III.

IF the tourist (to use a somewhat cockney
term) has not already been at Guildford, pray let
him or her take the first opportunity of doing
so.   It is a most interesting old place, scrupu-
lously clean, with quaint gable-roofed houses
and latticed windows, standing on the side of a
steep hill.   The old castle, the stage of many an
ancient historic scene from the earliest ages, is
chiefly of Norman architecture and full of
interest, and is well worth a visit.

Archbishop Abbot's hospital at the top of the
street, and the churches of the Holy Trinity
and St. Mary should be seen, especially the
latter.   In the Guildhall is a curious chimney-

piece in four compartments, representing ' Sanguineus,' 'Cholericus,' 'Phlegmaticus,' and ' Melancholicus.' All these ' lions ' should be visited with the aid of some good guide-book, but as our little work does not aspire to that dignity, I will leave the details to abler hands than mine.

Aubrey narrates an amusing story of Archbishop Abbot's rise in life. He was the son of a clothworker, and lived in a house adjoining the bridge. His mother, one night not long before his birth, dreamt that if she could have a jack or pike to eat, her child would rise to great distinction. Some time after, going to the river for water, she took up a jack in her pail, and in compliance with her dream, dressed and ate the fish. This circumstance becoming known in the neighbourhood, induced some influential people to offer themselves as sponsors, an offer which the poverty of the parents led them joyfully to accept. The sequel runs that as George Abbot and his brother Robert were playing one day on the bridge, some gentlemen, being struck with their appearance, and hearing of this curious dream, placed them at school, and subsequently sent them to the University, and in 1610 George was made archbishop of Canterbury. In the year 1621, the Archbishop had the mis-

fortune to kill Lord Zouch's keeper with an
arrow, whilst shooting at a deer in Bramshill
Park. This threw him into a deep melancholy,
and he kept a monthly fast ever afterwards on
the day of the week on which it happened; he
also settled an annuity of 40*l.* on the keeper's
widow.

The views from the tops of St. Catharine's and
St. Martha's hills, on which are situated chapels
of interest, are lovely, and in fact there are endless points in and around Guildford from whence
fine views are obtained. The old legend records
' that two sisters, Catharine and Martha, built
with their own hands the two chapels which
still bear their names. These ladies were of the
giant race, and the only working tool they used
was an enormous hammer, which they tossed
from one hill to the other as it was wanted.'

On the following morning we were up at seven,
and after a good breakfast, we commenced
foraging for supplies, and having procured some
meat pies (we need not pause to think of what
composed), we slipped our cable and glided under
the old bridge on our onward journey. The
inhabitants appeared to take great interest in
our proceedings, for the bridge was crowded with
spectators, and the little ' gamins ' of Guildford
ran along the towing-path after us for a long

distance. Our ardour here received a slight damper, for we beheld a small screw steamer which had just arrived from Brighton thoroughly disabled. We were informed that the weeds on the lower part of the Canal were so thick that she could scarcely make head against them, that they had completely fouled her screw, and to make bad worse, she had burst her boilers. We consoled ourselves, nevertheless, with the assurance that where the steamer could penetrate, we could do so too; moreover she must have opened a passage for herself, and thereby cleared a way for us.

Before leaving the town we borrowed from the boatman on the quay a ' new fangled ' implement with which to open the coming locks, called a winch; it was no doubt an immense improvement on our former weapon, for the locks on this Canal were to be opened from terra firma, and there was no further occasion to sit astride the gates, added to which the process of working the hatches was far easier, although, as this Canal is almost at a standstill from want of use, they were desperately stiff, and required at times all one's strength to open and shut.

After leaving Guildford we had still to pass the second lock with the aid of a crowbar, and we took a lad with us from the quay to take it back: it was a size larger than the one we had previously used. The scenery along this part is shut in by high hills, and the river winding its way along at their base, the *tout ensemble* has a very picturesque effect. Soon after passing the first lock we emerged into flat water-meadows, having St. Catharine's hill, crowned with its chapel, on our right, and the heights of Guildford and St. Martha's hill, beautifully wooded, behind us and on our left.

Here we met with our first serious check. On opening the lock we saw to our horror and dismay that there was scarcely a foot of water in the Canal. We pushed and punted along and carried away our towing rope in our efforts, and thus managed to gain about a hundred yards, when we stuck fast. What was to be done? we could neither get on nor back again, we could not land, for the mud was deep on either side of us, and we were fairly at our wits' end. In this dilemma we espied a woman making towards us. Our hopes instantly rose, as we thought she might be able to help us out of our difficulties. She commenced by informing us that we had no business where we were, that the water in that part of the Canal was let off for nine days to effect certain repairs to a mill on the Wey, and that meanwhile the lock-keepers

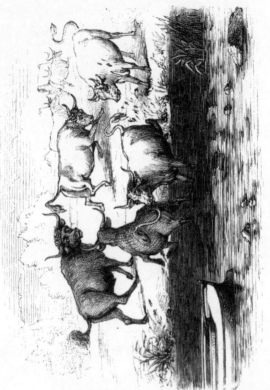

ALARMING POSITION.

had not the power to fill the Canal. She also told us that notices had been circulated to warn all barges and other craft, and that we ought to have been informed of this before we left Guildford.

We offered her anything to get us assistance, and we pleaded that we knew not the state of the water before we found ourselves stuck fast, that we only required about half a foot more to float us, and that a mile further on we should reach the next lock, where we should get into deep water again. The old lady there-upon became more amiable, and told us where a lock-keeper was to be found, who alone could help us in this disastrous emergency. We had, however, to send the groom on the pony in search of the man, who was at work about a mile off.

In the meantime we sat under umbrellas in the broiling sun, studying our journey and what was best to be done. At this juncture a large herd of formidable-looking oxen, having drawn them-selves up in line, charged down upon us with lowered heads and tails erect, threatening us with instant annihilation. I could fancy what the feelings of some of my fair friends would have been had they been obliged, as we were, to sit out this fierce charge. The animals however, on reaching the bank of our almost dried-up

Canal, seemed to be as much astonished as we were at finding it empty, and after snorting at us for some time as if chaffing at us in our ridiculous position, turned tail and charged back again to the other end of the field.

The man now made his appearance, and, after repeating what had been told us before, said he could get us more water, but that it would be a very expensive affair. After a while half-a-crown smoothed matters, and it occurred to him that he might be able to give us enough to get on with without flooding the works at the mill. He had, however, to go back to the lock above and let down the water for us, which obliged us to wait another half-hour.

By and by the joyful exclamation of 'here's the water' escaped our lips, and soon we found our little craft afloat again, and out of its difficulties once more. All these *contretemps* had detained us so long that we were very doubtful whether we could get on to Loxwood that night, which after Bramley was the only place where we could get board and lodging.

After passing through this shallow part, the canal flows under the railway bridge of the South Eastern, and at this point we took leave of the River Wey, which branches off to the right on its way to Godalming and Farnham. Here the

river deepened considerably, but immediately
after became even shallower than before, and we
had but just sufficient water to bring us into
the lock above, not however without much difficulty.   This junction of the Wey and the
Surrey and Sussex Canal is called Stonebridge,
taking its name from an old bridge which crosses
the canal just above.

The canal between Shalford, near Guildford
and Stonebridge, appears to be in different
hands, for we were here called upon to pay a toll
of one shilling, and right glad we were to find
ourselves in the Surrey and Sussex Canal.

This part of the country is uninteresting. The
Horsham and Guildford branch of the London,
Brighton and South Coast line runs along the
right bank; we presently came to a large tan-
yard on the left; and two more locks brought us
to Bramley.

At Bramley lock we made the acquaintance
of Mr. Stanton, the superintendent of the canal
at the Guildford end; he was most goodnatured
and gave us all the information we required,
besides offering us the run of his kitchen garden,
rich in gooseberries and currants.

The Surrey and Sussex Canal is worked by a
company, who procure the water from certain
reservoirs not far distant, and in dry summers

it frequently happens that the reservoirs cannot provide the necessary supply; the result
is that the whole navigation is at a standstill
until the next rains are good enough to start it
afresh; the company is therefore obliged to be
very particular that their water is not wasted.
They have in consequence laid down a rule that
no pleasure-craft of any sort is to pass through
their Canal without they have a bargee on
board who thoroughly understands the working
of the locks, and he is bound to shut them after
passing through, in order to keep the water up
as much as possible.

The Surrey and Sussex Canal forms the connecting link between the Rivers Wey and Arun,
thereby completing the through-navigation from
the sea at Littlehampton to the Thames at Weybridge. How long this connecting link will be
available seems most doubtful, for the whole of
this Canal is, I understand, to be put up immediately for auction. In fact, considering the
great expense in procuring water, the competi-
tion of the railway, and the small amount of
traffic, it is impossible it can pay its way. It
will be a sad pity if it ceases to exist, for the
scenery after leaving Bramley is most lovely,
and we thoroughly enjoyed our trip. The
original estimate for completing this Canal is
said to have been 71,000l.

Our little vessel being so small, we had not intended to proceed to sea in her until we reached Chichester harbour, for on examining the maps we found a Canal marked out between Ford, near Arundel, to Chichester harbour; this we had meant to use, and sailing from Chichester harbour, to come out into the Solent at Langston Harbour and Hayling Island.

Mr. Stanton (who I should mention is a coal merchant, and whose barges are constantly working through to Littlehampton) informed us to our dismay that this Canal no longer exists: in fact, there is now but small trace of it. He said it had not been used for eleven years, had been trodden in by cattle, filled-in in places, and was now quite dry. It behoved us, therefore, before proceeding further, to hold a council what was best to be done. Could we trust ourselves in our frail craft, which was only about half a foot above water, to the mercy of the waves round the headland of Selsea Bill and off the rough coast surrounding, or should we return to Guildford and put her on the train, giving up our contemplated trip further. We had serious doubts as to how our little vessel would behave in a sea-way, for we had never as yet been to sea in her, and to look at, she appeared but a cockle shell.

The various delays of this day had so run away with our time that we found it quite late before we reached Bramley, where we had to bait our pony and pull up for refreshment. We therefore agreed that it would be best not to try to get on further that day, as Loxwood was twelve miles ahead, with about twenty-one locks to open on the way. More time would be wanted to procure a bargee to accompany us, and we had not yet made up our minds whether or not to go on. After eating our luncheon, we took a stroll through the pretty little village of Bramley, and through a beautiful park, where we sat on the borders of a lake under the shade of the trees, watching a man catching bait with a casting net, and considering what would be our best course. At first we were averse to proceeding on our journey, as we did not wish to run any serious risk, which we might do were we to put to sea at Littlehampton: still the weather was fine, with a fair wind from the south-east, which made it very tempting. If, on the other hand, the weather should break up, and it became too rough for us to venture out to sea, we might be detained some time at Littlehampton, which would have been a serious inconvenience, for we were hurrying on to join a party to see the naval review at Spithead in honour of the Sultan.

We therefore decided on returning, and made the best of our way back to the lock. We lost no time in embarking, and set out on our return journey through the three locks to Stonebridge. We had, however, to get through the shallows again, and now there was not the excuse that we were ignorant that this part of the Canal was stopped, but we trusted that the water we should bring down through the lock, added to that which was given us in the morning, would be ample for our use. Alas! we were wrong; for, just after entering the shallow water, we stuck fast as a rock. We felt in a somewhat ridiculous position. Could we send for our friend a second time to get us more water? Would he not laugh us to scorn? Still we had nothing for it but to get hold of him again, and we therefore sent a lad to ferret him out. He was easily found this time, for he was busy haymaking not two fields off. We showed him another half-a-crown, and explained our case to him, and how we had found that the Arundel and Portsmouth Canal was a myth. After some parley he set off to shut the lower lock, which he had opened to let the water off after we had passed up in the morning. All this occupied about an hour, during which time we sat in our boat lamenting the necessity of having to put back. At this moment a bargee passing by cried out, ' Halloa, sir, I thought you were bound for Littlehampton.' He was a man to whom we had spoken in the morning, and who had been anxious to go with us through the locks. When we told him our predicament, he strongly advised us to persevere, assuring us that we should have fine weather, with a calm sea, round Selsea Bill. As it required but a feather to turn the scale, this set us thinking again—had we not better go on ? The toss of a half-a-crown settled the point, for ' heads ' was the cry, which we had arranged should be for proceeding; it fell ' heads ' just as the additional water reached us. We entered Stone-bridge lock for the third time, determined that nothing should now send us back again. In process of time we got to Bramley once more, much to the surprise of Mr. Stanton and the natives. It was too late to proceed farther that day, so we deposited our goods in safe keeping in Mr. Stanton's stores, and set out in search of a dinner and a lodging for the night.

We were advised to try the Grantley Arms at Wonersh, a village on the left of the canal, about half a mile distant. We set off to mount the hill, followed by the groom and pony. On arriving at the Grantley Arms, we found it a pokey little inn where of course we could get no accommodation, so back we had to come to try our luck at Bramley. This was still worse, and we began to doubt whether we should ever find rooms for the night.

But the old saying 'never say die' held good in our case, for in our search we had to pass by the railway station, where we noticed a crowd of people evidently waiting for a train. The idea at once struck us, 'Let us go where the train will take us, and return in the morning.' On inquiry, to our joy, we heard a train for Guildford was then due, and giving instructions to the groom to get a bed at the Bramley inn, and a stall for the pony, we got into the train, and started back to Guildford.

We put up for the night at the White Hart, in my opinion the best hotel in Guildford, where we regaled ourselves with a capital dinner, and were thankful that we were not in the Grantley Arms at Wonersh.

CHAPTER IV.

ARRANGEMENTS FOR OUR ONWARD JOURNEY—SCENERY ABOUT
BRAMLEY—GATES IN THE TOWING PATH—WEALD OF SURREY
—LOXWOOD — THE FISHERMAN — WEEDS IN THE CANAL —
GEORGE COX, THE BARGEE—ARRIVAL AT NEWBRIDGE—BIL-
LINGHURST—THE 'KING'S ARMS'—THE CHURCH—ARRANGE-
MENTS FOR THE MORROW.

THE following morning we left Guildford for
Bramley by the 7·20 train, which got us there
in about a quarter of an hour.   Our groom was
waiting for us at the station, and we at once
despatched him to fetch the pony, whilst we
made the best of our way down to the locks.
There we found a bargee lad, George Cox by
name, about nineteen years of age, whom Mr.
Stanton had procured to pioneer us through the
locks, armed with his own 'winch,' which ena-
bled me to return the one lent to us by the
boatman at Guildford.

Before starting, Mr. Stanton demanded a
toll of 5s. from us for our way bill to Newbridge,
the terminus of the Surrey and Sussex Canal
Company, and we got off at about 8·30 *en route*

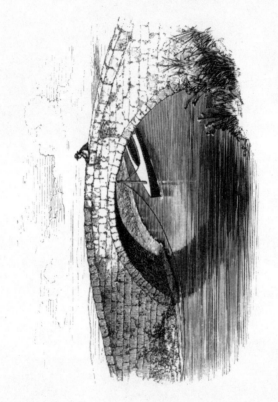

LOW BRIDGES.

for Loxwood and Billinghurst, at the latter of which places we proposed to halt for the night.

The scenery, immediately on quitting Bramley, becomes lovely, and we were still blessed with the most splendid weather. The Canal winds its way under the shade of woods on each side, which come quite down to the water's edge, where the water-lilies, both white and yellow, were floating in profusion. The birds were singing most energetically, as if to make up for lost time during the past wet and cold spring and summer, and the little moor-hens ducked under water, with wild screams on all sides, as we approached. We here passed through the property of Lord Grantley (Green Place). The lowest of bridges span the Canal at intervals, under some of which our mast almost shaved the top, and we had to be most careful to steer for the very centre of the arches.

It was most fortunate that I had had the towing-mast reduced from eight to seven feet in length before starting, for had it been one inch higher, we should have been obliged to unship it at every bridge we came to. From time to time, we had to open small iron drawbridges; but we got on this day much faster than before, for our pioneer, knowing what was coming, could

D

always run ahead to prepare the way for us. He was a most energetic youth, and, in spite of the intense heat of a broiling sun, would rush from one lock to the other at a great pace.

The swing-gates, which had hitherto impeded our progress, tormented us even more on this day; for the provoking people, not content with single gates, had made them double, so that it was now impossible to ride through them; and at almost every field, the groom had to dismount to free the towing-rope, causing considerable delay.

After enjoying this delicious cool shade for a distance of about two miles, we were forced to brave the scorching rays of a morning sun. It was well for us that we had started early, for the sun had not yet reached its full power; and we had to pass through about five miles of flat open heathery common and water-meadows, before again entering into a charming country—the well-known Weald of Surrey. Murray tells us that we should traverse a portion of this Weald country, with its fine old farmhouses, relics of the prosperous old times of the Weald; its old ponds, vestiges of the many iron furnaces of former days; its old families of yeomen and labourers, and wide-stretching oak plantations, still maintaining for it something of its primal character. Cobbett says of the real Weald of Surrey, that it is ' a country where, strictly speaking, only three things will grow well—grass, wheat, and oak-trees.'

Into these beautiful oak plantations we now entered by a perfectly straight and deep cutting, about a mile and a half in length, with numbers of low stone bridges crossing the Canal at intervals, which presented a very striking effect. It is from these highlands that many of the tributaries of the Rivers Wey and Arun spring—Hindhead, not many miles distant, being the watershed of this district.

Our route now lay through a most refreshing and picturesque country of a broken and undulating character, densely clothed with a forest of oak-trees, opening out and giving peeps into deep hollows verdant with luxuriant ferns and purple heather. Here and there were breaks in the woodland, and the small round hills, rich in pasturage, appeared—the ancient folds of the Weald.

We now commenced to make our descent towards the sea, and lock after lock followed each other in rapid succession, there being no less than eleven in one mile. Soon after passing through the last, we arrived at Loxwood at about 1.30 P.M. Here we made our midday halt, and whilst the pony was resting, we sat in the shade of a big oak, regaling ourselves with the good fare we had brought with us. Loxwood is a small place, but boasts of a neat clean little inn close by the Canal-side; and I think I might safely recommend it for sleeping quarters, although, being early in the day, we did not pull up here, but pressed forward to Billinghurst.

Whilst I was quietly enjoying my pipe after lunch, my curiosity was raised by seeing a man amusing himself throwing a large stone into the Canal attached to a long line, which he hauled in and flung back over and over again. On approaching him, I soon discovered his little dodge, for I beheld a number of small branches floating about in all directions, to which fine gut-lines and hooks were attached, wherewith to ensnare the wily fish, somewhat on the principle of the trimmer. These boughs he got to land by means of his stone, which he flung over them, drawing them slowly ashore. I did not see him catch anything, although I watched him for some time; but he assured me he had been very successful by this plan, and had at times secured pike and other fish of a large size.

At 3 P.M. we started again on our way to Billinghurst, five miles distant from Loxwood, and seventeen from Bramley. There are five locks between Loxwood and Newbridge.

The country here is decidedly ugly, with flat water-meadows on either side. The Canal at this point became exceedingly weedy, and I was obliged to stand 'forward,' to clear the bows from the weeds which clung to her. Just before reaching Newbridge they became so thick that it seemed almost impossible to cut our way through them, and this was the spot where the steamer we had seen at Guildford had come to grief.

At Newbridge Lock our pilot, George Cox, left us. We paid him his fee of 10s., and he returned to Bramley. He had been very civil, and most active and energetic, and was of the greatest assistance to us. If any of my readers undertake this trip, from the Thames to the sea by Canal, they could not do better than engage this young fellow's services from Bramley to Newbridge. About a mile below the lock we came to Newbridge (a fine stone bridge), where we brought up for the day. It was about 5.30 P.M., and it took some little time to collect our goods together, anchor our craft, and clean and stow everything away safely.

Immediately upon our arrival, we despatched the groom on the pony to Billinghurst, a dis-

tance of almost one mile and a half, to secure
rooms and a dinner for us, and after getting all
ship-shape on board, we ourselves started for
the village.

The road led us uphill, through a rich open
country highly cultivated; and on our right
was the range of the South Downs, with the
well-known Danish encampment of Chancton-
bury Ring, where I (and I have no doubt many
others) have often spent a jolly day picnicking.

In the Saxon language Hurst means a 'wood:'
thus Brockenhurst signifies the 'wood of the
badger,' Lyndhurst the 'linden wood,' Holden-
hurst the 'grove of oaks,' &c. &c.   Billinghurst, therefore, means Billing's wood,
Billing being the name of a great Saxon tribe.
The village of Billinghurst lies on the Roman
Stane Street which ran from Chichester to London, Billingsgate being probably the end of the
road.   We found it a charming little place,
with a neat clean inn, 'The King's Arms;' and
having secured our rooms and changed our
attire, we had the gratification of sitting down
to as good a dinner as, I believe, it is possible
to get in a quiet country village.   Everything
was fresh and good of its kind; eggs, butter,
bread, fruit, cream, all excellent; and our mut-
ton-chops done to a turn, with excellent beer
and very fair sherry.

After dinner we took a stroll up the village. It was a lovely evening, and all seemed peaceful and happy: little family groups sitting at the entrance-doors of their houses, others strolling up and down the hilly street, while the young ones besported themselves on all sides. Judging from the appearance of the old men we saw crawling about in every direction, the place must be most healthy, which doubtless is the case; for it stands on high ground, and appeared beautifully clean and thriving. Billinghurst Church is worth a visit; the south side is very Early Norman, the rest Perpendicular.

Before retiring for the night we had to make arrangements for the morrow, as we were anxious to start very early, in order, if possible, to press on to Littlehampton the same evening: added to which, on approaching the sea, we had to consider the tides, which would first reach us at Waltham Lock—the last lock on our journey, about three miles above Amberley. We found that the tide ebbed at Waltham at 12 P.M., so that, in order to get there on the first of the ebb, it was necessary that we should make an early start from Billinghurst. We consequently contrived to persuade our good landlady to have us called at 5 A.M., and to have a breakfast ready for us by a quarter to 6.

CHAPTER V.

THERE are some favoured individuals (amongst whom I am glad to number myself) who have the power of calling themselves at whatever hour of the morning they wish to awake, thereby rendering themselves quite independent. True enough, at 4.30 I awoke and roused the house; it was a first-class morning, such as few of the 'Upper Ten Thousand' often see. It is a sad pity that human nature requires so much slumber, for everyone seems to want a certain number of hours, short of which they are apt to feel out of sorts, and not quite up to the mark : were it otherwise, and would the customs of our time admit of our not turning night into day, especially in the summer, I am sure that much pleasure would be found in the delicious freshness of those early morning hours.

After a bit the little inn was in a bustle—hot and cold water for shaving, and baths, to any amount, and boots polished like mirrors; thus our toilettes were accomplished with as much comfort as if we had been *chez nous.* I can fancy my readers saying, 'Well done—that sounds like business!' So it was, but we have not done yet. The breakfast was a capital one, and as punctual as we could wish; for our little table saw its cold meat, eggs, toast, and coffee awaiting us at the given hour of 5.45 A.M.

The bill was very moderate, and we all got off at 6.30. A little before 7 o'clock we reached Newbridge, where our boat lay quietly at her moorings, wet with her morning bath of dew. It took us but a short time to get under way, and 'Forward!' was the cry. The bargees and lockmen had informed us, the day before, that we need not encumber ourselves with crowbar or winch, for we should find them at the locks *pro bono publico.*

The same meadow-scenery continued, and the same lovely weather. In about an hour's time we reached the first lock, which was opened for us whilst we watched the lock-keeper's wife and two pretty daughters making butter in the early morn. Though flat, the meadows no each side presented such a truly English picture

—with cattle dotted about here and there and in groups, the larks soaring aloft sending forth their melodious morning song, and the banks of the Canal clothed with wild flowers of every hue and colour—that we enjoyed this part of our route almost as much as any. The Canal, after leaving Newbridge, becomes much narrower, and the locks are considerably smaller, with single instead of double gates : this part of it, from Newbridge to Pallingham, is in different hands, and is said to have cost 15,000*l.*

We had about three locks to pass before we arrived at the great Pallingham Lock, which is the largest I ever saw—about 40 feet long and 30 feet deep, and wide enough for two good-sized barges to lie alongside each other. The lock-keeper was not at home, so I had to fill this great basin single-handed, which was no joke, for it required a considerable amount of strength. Here was the receiving-house of the Arun Canal Company, where we were called upon to pay a shilling toll. The lock-keeper's wife made tender enquiries after the steamer we had seen at Guildford. It had passed up two days previously, and the good lady had not heard of the accident which befell it.

A short distance after passing through Pallingham Lock, we entered the River Arun, which was considerably wider than the Canal, so that our towing-rope became too short, and we were obliged to make use of the boat's cable, which we made fast to the end of it.

The Arun's source is in St. Leonard's Forest, and the river is celebrated for its mullet, trout, and eels. We now observed a striking contrast between canal and river travelling. The banks of the Canal, although in places excessively pretty, were almost always perfectly parallel, and presented a certain artificial formality which does not exist in the natural river. The Arun's banks, on the contrary, were varied— now steep, now broken and low ; and at times the towing-line had to pass over the tops of tall sedges and alders, the river being now wide, now narrow, now deep, now shallow—for ever varying.

Our course lay through a fine park, with likely-looking coverts dotted all around, from which, no doubt, many a pheasant has fallen a victim, and many a fox has been unkenneled. We saw the keeper and his dogs crossing the park, which looked as if there was, or ought to be, game on the property, and I have no doubt good fishing and boating in the Arun besides. On leaving the park, we came under a picturesque

old stone bridge to Stopham. There is an inn
close to the river, where a halt might be made
to see the old church, which is interesting and
of Norman architecture; there is also a fine
view over the Weald country, from a hill at the
back of the village.

The river now winds a good deal through
water-meadows, in the midst of which we
arrived at the junction of the Arun with the
Rother, which latter river is navigable to
Midhurst, and under the management of the
Arun Canal Company. We are told that this
company still pays its way, and that, before the
railroad was opened, it was in a flourishing
state, producing a very comfortable dividend.

We soon came to Hardham Lock and Mill.
Whilst the lock was filling, I entered into con-
versation with a gentleman, who I soon found
out was Mr. Frank Buckland. He had come
down from London, with five or six other
Commissioners, to inspect the capabilities of
the river for salmon-fishing. They seemed to
take great interest in our proceedings, and
Mr. Buckland produced his Ordnance Map, and
begged me to point out to him the route we had
traversed. Whilst we were thus busily engaged,
the groom hallooed out, 'Look out, sir!—
look out!' We at once discovered that the

boat had drifted under an iron footbridge which crossed the lock; and as the water rose, she began to settle down deeper and deeper—the mast being wedged so firmly under the bridge that we could not get it free. I rushed to stop the water coming in, and opened the hatches at the other end. In the meanwhile, Mr. Buckland very kindly stood by the side of the lock, to render any assistance my wife might require in this critical position. It was fortunate that we had discovered our predicament in time, for the water was almost level with the bulwarks of the boat before it commenced to decrease, and a little more would have caused her to fill.

About a couple of hundred yards from this spot, the river makes a détour of about five miles round by Pulborough, to avoid which a canal has been cut, passing through the chalk cliff by means of a tunnel. At the entrance of this tunnel we found another small lock, where we parted company with the pony, which had to go over the top, and meet us at the other end. This tunnel is a quarter of a mile long, 13 feet wide, the same in height, and cost 6,000*l.* I punted the boat along by means of the boat-hook against the roof. In the middle it became quite dark, and we could only just guide ourselves by means of the bright outlet at the end.

The roof was covered with stalactites, and in
places the water fell upon us from crevices
above in heavy drops, so that we had to try
and steer clear of them where we heard their
splashes on the water below. It took about
ten minutes to pass through this subterranean
passage, and when we emerged on the other side,
it was some moments before we became accustomed to the bright light of day. We were
detained here some little while, for the groom
had mistaken his way, and did not turn up for
about twenty minutes after we got out of the
tunnel. We recommenced our journey along a
flat country, still in the Canal, until we reached
Waltham Lock at about 12.30 P.M., where we
found that the tide had, as we calculated, just
begun to ebb.

It was with a feeling of satisfaction that we
now found ourselves in a tideway at no great distance from the sea. The tide had turned about
half an hour before we got to Waltham, the last
lock on our journey, and the river began to
shoal in many parts. It also became very wide,
and we had about 100 yards of towing-line out
at one time, and were going at a brisk pace, when
we were suddenly brought up.

We had come to an aggravating kind of gate.
The principle upon which it worked was inge-

THE TUNNEL.

nious in itself, but it seemed to have been made
to puzzle people's brains as to how they should
pass it. It consisted of two upright posts in the
ground, with three wooden bars fixed across
them, each working upon a pivot, and weighted
at one end; so that, in order to open the gate, it
was necessary to press the bars down to the
ground, and hold them in that position until the
animal had stepped over, when, by letting them
go, the weighted end fell, and the bars sprung
back into a horizontal position.* This may be all
very well where two persons are present, the one
to lead the beast over while the other presses
down the bars; but how one alone is to get on,
with a timid or fidgetty animal, it is difficult to
say. We had encountered one or two of these
gates before on this day's journey, but the pony
had always willingly stepped over them whilst
the groom held the bars down; but on this occasion, in doing so, they accidentally sprang up
under her, while she was in the act of clearing
them, which frightened her to such a degree that
no persuasion would induce her to attempt to
cross them again.

The groom tried every artifice he could devise
to get her over: he tied the bars down, got on
her back, and rode at them, coaxed her—but all

* See Illustration, page 59

in vain!   Meanwhile we could render no assistance, for we were in the centre of a wide tidal river, with steep mud banks on each side of us, where there were no means of landing. It was evident, however, that I *must* land somehow or other, to help; so away we paddled with the sweeps, in the hopes of being able to find a landing place. We fortunately succeeded about a quarter of a mile below, where I got ashore as best I could, and ran back to the groom, whom I found still labouring to get the pony over the gate. We tried all kinds of dodges without avail: at last I had resort to whipping her over while he led her at it, and she ultimately cleared it as though she were going at a five-barred gate.

Away we went again, and soon picked up the boat; but we had lost, sad to say, nearly an hour's tide. Two or three of the same kind of fences followed each other, at which we had more or less difficulty, and we did not reach Amberley until nearly two o'clock. Here we brought up, to make our midday halt.

Let us pause at this stage for a short time, to examine the interesting ruins of Amberley Castle.

The castle is constructed on a rock, and is in the form of a parallelogram having a square tower at each corner. The exterior wall in the north is the most perfect, then the east and west ends, but the south is not in such good preservation. It is defended on this side by a fosse, over which a bridge leads to the principal entrance between two small round towers, with grooves for a portcullis. On the north and west sides it appears to have been of no great strength: the ruins of an arch within the walls prove the architecture to have been light and elegant. Amberley Castle was used as a residence by the Bishops of Chichester from the time of the Conquest. It was castellated in 1379. In 1643, after the surrender of Arundel Castle, it also fell into the hands of Cromwell's troops, who plundered and dismantled it without mercy.

The little church which adjoins is also well worth visiting. The chancel is Norman, and the south door very rich Early English.

The Amberley sea-trout are famous, though not very plentiful.

But we must not delay longer, or we shall lose our tide, especially as one mile farther down the river, at a place called Houghton, the towing path comes to an end, and we must there take to our oars for a seven-miles' pull to Arundel. Wishing, however, to give the pony a good rest after her long morning's work, we

E

commenced to row at once. The tide was running strong when we passed under the old bridge at Amberley, eating our luncheon as we drifted on. We went by Bury Hill at a great pace, and soon came to the overhanging wooded cliffs of Arundel Park. The river is here strikingly pretty, and we met a great number of pleasure boats rowing and fishing. We thoroughly enjoyed this enchanting scene, and did not hurry ourselves, when, all at once, it occurred to us that the tide was getting slacker. We asked a boatman, who seemed to be hurrying on, how far it was to Arundel. He replied, ' Oh, a long way, if you don't make haste, you won't get there to-day.' This sounded very discouraging, as we knew that, should the tide turn, it would be impossible for us to row against it for any distance; no time was therefore to be lost, so we set to work and pulled our best.

We soon left the shelter of the woods, the river winding out into the plain, with high mud banks on each side of us, covered with extensive beds of tall-growing sedges. The tide soon began to work up the centre of the river, and we had to hug the banks to try and cheat it. It was now becoming hard work, and we had still a long way before us—it was impossible to get out and tow, for the soft mud-

banks at low water were deep and high, even
where they were clear of rushes. We had
therefore to stick to our work, each pulling in
turn, and sometimes both together. By and
bye we came to a point where one branch of
the river led off to the left, and the other went
straight on—in our maps the straight course
was not indicated, and the one to the left was
marked as leading to Stoke, by which we
afterwards found we should have had to follow
three or four great bends of the river before
reaching Arundel. After a minute's consulta-
tion, we thought we would chance the course
which led straight on, and right glad we were
that we had done so, for it certainly shortened
our distance by two or three miles. At last the
Castle opened to view, this gave us fresh energy,
and we pulled right well. In about another
hour we met some barges coming up with the
tide, they told us we had only about one mile
more, and that we could easily get on the same
evening to Littlehampton. This was good
news, and a reward for our perseverance, especially as we had by this time quite made up
our minds that we should be obliged to stop the
night at Arundel, thinking it impossible to
reach Littlehampton that evening against a
strong tide ; added to which about a hundred

yards ahead we espied our groom running
along the water-meadows to meet us; he had
fetched our letters, which we had desired our
friends to address to Arundel. We flung him
a towing rope, and made him pull us up to the
bridge, where we arrived at about 5·30 P.M.
He then left us to fetch the pony; meanwhile
we had a stiff job to get the boat through the
bridge, for the tide was now rushing up like a
sluice. We made several attempts, but were
beaten; at last we got close to the wall, and
pulled ourselves through by means of the boat-
hook, and so all along the sides of the houses
which, with the quays, present one even face
to the river. After getting below the town, the
tide slackened a little, and we here awaited
the arrival of the pony.

The word Arundel is said to be a *liaison*
between the words Arun and Hirondelle. A
steep street leads from the river to the castle.
Tickets are issued at the hotel to see the keep
and grounds, but the inhabited part of the
castle is not shown. The first mention of
Arundel is made in the will of Alfred the
Great. Tradition states that Bevis was the
founder of the castle, and there still exists a
tower called Bevis' tower. Gilpin says, 'Bevis
was a giant of ancient times, whose power was

equal to his size. He was able to wade the channel of the sea to the Isle of Wight, and frequently did it for his amusement. Great, however, as Bevis was, he condescended to be warder at the gate of the Earls of Arundel, who built this tower for his reception, and supplied him with two hogsheads of beer every week, a whole ox, and a proportional quantity of bread and mustard. It is true the dimensions of the tower are only proportioned to a man of moderate size, but such an inconsistence is nothing when opposed to the traditions of a country.'

Earl Roger de Montgomery and his sons successively held it until 1118, when it was granted by Henry I. to his Queen Adeliza, who married William de Albini. It is related that before his marriage the Queen of France, a woman of great beauty, being then a widow, caused a tournament to be proclaimed throughout her dominions. On this occasion Albini repaired to Paris, and bore away the palm from all his competitors. The Queen, struck with the prowess and person of the champion, invited him to an entertainment, and having presented him with some jewels of great value, made him an offer of her hand. Having already engaged his word to Adeliza, he declined this splendid match, on which the Queen, as we are told, to revenge the disappointment, ordered him to be shut up in a lion's den, where the undaunted Albini, thrusting his hand into the mouth of the formidable brute, pulled up his tongue by the roots. From this action he is said to have acquired the appellation of William-with-the-Strong-Hand.

The Empress Maud was the guest of Queen Adeliza when she came over to dispute her claims with King Stephen. The King having heard of her presence in the castle, besieged it, and demanded her surrender. Queen Adeliza sent him a spirited message to the effect that ' She had received the Empress as her friend, not as his enemy, and that, as she did not intend to mix herself up in these disputes, she begged that the Empress might be allowed to depart, but,' she added, ' if you are determined to besiege her here, I will endure the last extremity of war rather than give her up, or suffer the laws of hospitality to be violated.' King Stephen assented and the Empress retired to Bristol.

In 1243 the estates went by marriage to the Fitzalans. ' It is said that Richard, Earl of Arundel, was accused of conspiring with others against the life of King Richard II. He was tried and condemned. The King was present at his execution, and the spectacle remained so deeply imprinted on his mind, that his sleep was interrupted by dreams representing to him the Earl covered with blood, and upbraiding him with his injustice. A rumour prevailed that several miracles were wrought at his tomb, and that his head was miraculously rejoined to his body. To counteract this notion, the King ordered the corpse to be taken up and exposed for ten successive days to public view. Still nothing could persuade the people that the Earl was not a martyr. Nothing could be more unpopular than the execution of this nobleman, who possessed many valuable qualities, had served with great success against the enemy, and always asserted the liberties of the people, by whom he was much beloved.'

The Fitzalans held the castle and estates till 1580, when Earl Fitzalan's daughter inheriting it, brought it by marriage to the house of Norfolk.

Arundel Castle underwent three sieges, the first in 1102 by Henry I., again by Stephen, and in December, 1643, by the Parliamentary troops under Sir W. Waller, to whom it surrendered. It is said that during the last siege, artillery played upon it from the church steeple, which reduced the greater part to ruins.

The keep is the principal sight to see, and is

well worth a visit. From the top of it there is
a splendid view, and the Isle of Wight and
Chichester Cathedral are to be seen on a clear
day. The great hobby of the ancestors of the
present Duke appears to have been a large collection of sea-owls, which bred in the ivy towers
of the keep, the whole of which was covered in
by netting, to prevent their taking flight. Some
of these birds are now to be seen stuffed, and
they appear each to have had its name. An
amusing story is told of one, which they called
' Lord Thurlow.' Whilst a large party were at
dinner in the castle, the attendants rushed in
with joy on their countenances, exclaiming :
' Grand news ! Lord Thurlow's laid an egg.'
This celebrated bird, with the identical egg (?),
is still to be seen in the collection at the keep.

The church at Arundel also contains some fine
monuments, but the Great Park is perfectly
charming : we had been here not long before, and
I still remember how we enjoyed our wanderings
in the glades, valleys, and heights of this lovely
spot. I could not pass this grand old castle
without alluding to its glories, and as we glided
by, it was not without a lingering wish to stay
and have another look at it.

The last stage of our journey to the sea now
commenced. We had, as I have before nar-

rated, encountered great trouble in overcoming the obstacles in the shape of gates above Arundel, and had congratulated ourselves they were passed, when we came upon a long line of them, which, we were informed by a gentleman who helped us over the first, continued all the way to Littlehampton.

He suggested that we should try the plan generally found to answer by the bargemen, viz. to blindfold the animal, but this was of no avail, and rather made matters worse.

Sussex was always famous for its ingenious gates, but this three-barred arrangement beats anything one ever saw; they seemed to find favour with no one, for all whom we met abused them, and they gave us endless trouble. At last we discovered the quickest plan was to lead the pony to the gate, the bars being fastened down, then to lift one leg over and place it firmly on the ground on the opposite side, and so coax her over. By means of these and other dodges we progressed on our way. The tide was strong against us, but the pony was still stronger, so we quickly went ahead.

The appearance of the river now showed us we were evidently approaching the sea. Its great width, the shipping in the distance, and the number of small craft of every description dotted about—some busy fishing, some anchored, some under sail—presented a very animated appearance.

Soon after passing Ford the town began to appear, and in about twenty minutes we came to the end of the towing path, which brought us into the heart of the river. We had been cautioned against the chains of the floating bridge, which stretch across the river under water, and it was just at the point where the pony's good services ceased, that we came upon the bridge in question.

It was then about 8·30 P.M. and getting dark. The good man who minded the ferry, a thick-set handsome fellow and evidently a good seaman, recommended us, after hearing our story, to put up at a new little inn kept by a pal of his facing the harbour, opposite to the place where we had brought up. The Beach Hotel, the great house of the place, was a mile and a half further on, and as we were anxious to get our dinner as soon as possible, and to procure information with respect to our first attempt on the high seas, as well as to get hold of a respectable sailor capable of piloting us to Portsmouth, we left our craft for the night in the charge of the ferryman, and proceeded to the little inn on the opposite side of the river.

OBNOXIOUS GATES.

The good lady of the house and her charming daughter exerted themselves to their utmost to make us comfortable; they gave us a prettily furnished sitting room, having a bay window looking out upon the harbour, from whence we could see our little ship lying at anchor amongst the schooner and cutter-yachts, a proud position for her.

Previous to going to dinner, I had commissioned my friend the ferryman to find me a pilot, and to send him to me at the inn. As soon as dinner was concluded I was informed of his presence, and he was accordingly ushered in. He appeared somewhat unsteady on his pins, and one could scarcely say he had got his sea-legs. After informing him that I required some competent man to pilot us to Portsmouth, and consulting with him as to the weather and the coast, he hummed and hawed a good deal, and said that he did not much like the job, that he had been out all day fishing off Selsea Bill, and that there had been a nasty lumpy sea which would be almost too much for our boat, and that he could not think of undertaking the 'voyage' with a lady aboard. This did not sound very promising, particularly as the lady had no sort of intention of being left behind, so we told him he had better think over it, and we would see how the weather looked in the morning. Later in the evening, whilst I was enjoying my nocturnal pipe, I came across the ferryman again, who thought the skipper must be an idiot, for with fair wind and tide we should only take about six hours to reach Portsmouth, and he said that he only wished that he could get time from his duty to go with us.

In this state of uncertainty we went to roost, ordering them to call us at six o'clock in the morning.

CHAPTER VI.

To our infinite joy, the following morning dawned as bright as its predecessors, with the wind north-east and a nice sailing breeze. No- thing could be more fortunate. We were up be- times, thinking it probable we might find some difficulty in securing the services of a competent individual to sail with us to the Solent. To our great surprise and delight, on looking from the window we saw the little vessel's bergee flying at her masthead, and her mainsail partly set, which proved that the skipper, having slept over his stern decision of the night before, had made up his mind to sail with us after all.

We now despatched the groom and pony to their destination by road, a distance of about 40 miles, having no further need of their services.

After breakfast we set to work to procure refreshments in case we might require them, and to repair any little losses we had sustained *en route*. An hour sufficed to put all in order, and at 9 A.M. we weighed anchor and proceeded to beat out of the harbour. Under the lighthouse there was a little broken sea, which made us think we should catch it outside, but the boat was so buoyant and behaved so well, that we did not ship a drop of water. After proceeding about two miles out to procure an offing, we laid our course parallel with the shore, the breeze was steady and fresh, and we spun along with a fair tide at about eight knots an hour. A sense of freedom and rest stole over us as we bounded merrily over the waves, delighted at the successful performance of the boat, which more than answered our expectations, and we were but too glad we had not put back at Bramley.

No more locks to open; no more aggravating gates to pass; nothing to prevent me lying down in my plaids, and smoking my pipe in peace, whilst the winds and the waves did all the work for us. Our trip by canal had been quite charming, but rather hard work, and after our four days' labour, we were glad of the change.

We soon passed the towns of Middleton and

Bognor, with their explanades and white-fronted houses lighted up by the sun, and giving Pagham harbour a wide berth, we steered a little out to weather the point of Selsea Bill.

In process of time we arrived off the point, a bleak wild shore, bearing most unmistakably the marks of the ravages of storm and tempest. In the early Saxon times, Selsea was peopled by a heathen race, who lived from hand to mouth as best they could. This district was granted by the king to Bishop Wilfred, who founded the see (since removed to Chichester) and built a cathedral and monastery there. On his arrival he found the people in sad distress, for Bede tells us they had had no rain for three years, and were plunged into the most abject poverty, destroying themselves in numbers to avoid starvation. On the first day of baptism, however, the rain fell heavily, and the aspect of affairs changed for the better. There is at present no trace whatever of the cathedral or monastery, all no doubt having been destroyed by the inroads of the sea. The anchorage to the eastward of the bill, still called the park, was stocked with deer in the days of Bluff King Hal, when many a good haunch of venison found its way without doubt to the table of the monastery.

The village of Selsea is about half a mile from the shore: how long that will stand, 'who can tell?'

On rounding the point, we espied in the distance the Channel Fleet in 'beauteous order ranged.' It was a most imposing sight, these magnificent ships, all getting up their steam for a rehearsal preparatory to the grand review. We unanimously decided to sail out of our course in the direction of St. Helen's Roads, where the fleet lay at anchor. It was not long before we reached them, and it was a grand sight to see them get under way with the greatest possible precision, and glide through the sea, side by side, almost without one's being aware that they were in motion. We watched their evolutions for some time, and perceived that one of the ironclads had carried away her jib-boom, and appeared as though she had already been engaged with the enemy.

Our attention was so wrapped up in the movements of the fleet, that we had not noticed that the wind had been freshening to a very great extent, and that we had left the shore about 14 miles astern, the sea in the meantime having risen considerably. It therefore became necessary for us at once to shape our course for Portsmouth, and in order to do so, we must gibe the sail. The skipper, unaccustomed to boats of this rig, appealed to me to say how this was to be done with the strong breeze then blowing. I informed him that he was as wise as I was, for that this was my first trip to sea in the ' Caprice.' I told him I thought we had nothing to fear if we gibed the sail carefully. He however, on consideration, thought it would be safer to 'stay' her, considering the large size of her single sail. I was very doubtful as to the advisability of this course, for in coming round we must present a broadside to the rollers, which were running high at the time, and if we then by accident shipped a sea, the probabilities were that we should be swamped, added to which I had always been told that these Una boats were good for nothing in a sea-way. Nevertheless I yielded to the superior knowledge of the 'skipper,' and we 'went about.' She came round very gamely, rising like a duck to the waves. Before, however, we could put her before the wind, a great roller charged us broadside on, breaking over her, and giving us a good ducking, which obliged us to set to work to bale out.

We now went ahead at a great pace towards Portsmouth; the rollers threatening to poop us all the time, but we were going too fast for

them, and at about 2 P.M. we dropt anchor in
front of Southsea pier.

We landed in a shore-boat which came out
to us, and having discharged our pilot, we
proceeded at once to the Queen's Hotel, where
we did ample justice to a good luncheon; after
which we started for Cumberland Fort, to visit
some friends quartered there. They very kindly
showed us over the new barracks built for the
Marine Artillery. Nothing can be more perfect than their arrangement. A large area is
covered in, under which the troops drill in bad
weather, leading into which, all round, are the
several rooms appropriated to the use of the
officers and men. Reading rooms, libraries,
mess rooms, billiard and gymnastic rooms, lec-
ture rooms, &c., &c., as comfortable and snug
as in a London club. The dormitories, lava-
tories, washhouses—all in the most perfect
style. Indeed, the wonder is, that every man
who enlists does not join the Royal Marine
Artillery. The houses appropriated to the
married officers are not yet finished. We were
told that each would have a house to himself
when ready. They face the sea, and are built
upon the open drill ground of the regiment.
We were shown guns mounted in every position for gun drill; one of which was placed

upon a stage, and made to rise and fall by means of machinery, to imitate the motion of a vessel at sea. The men have also their out-door amusements, for any of them who wish it may try their hands at horticulture, and have a small plot each allotted to him for that pur-pose. We walked through these little gardens, and it was curious to see the British marines, dressed in their uniforms, hard at work digging and raking their respective plots.

At 5·30 P.M., we left the fort accompanied by our friends, who were anxious to see us off, and to have a look at the 'Caprice.' The fort is three miles from the pier, so that it took us nearly half an hour to get there.

On our way we came in for a beautiful sight. The fleet, which we had watched in the morning manœuvring under steam, was now returning to Spithead under a full press of canvas, which had a very grand effect, and it was excessively interesting to watch these great ships each drop into her respective place, and then at once come to an anchor.

We were put on board our little craft by a shore-boat, and were soon off again on our way to Ryde. Our course lay straight through the fleet, and we delayed some time cruizing in and out to obtain a nearer view of some of

them. We had tickets to admit us on board one
of the Peninsula and Oriental steamers, char-
tered by the government on the day of the
review, but as the weather on that occasion did
not permit of the fleet performing any evolutions, we saw it to much greater advantage on
this day, although nothing could be grander
than the splendid cannonade which took place
at the review.

The ships were anchored in two parallel lines,
the wooden on one side and the ironclads on the
other; the wooden ships looking by far the most
formidable, although there was a rakish kind
of aspect about the ironclads, as though they
did not intend to be trifled with, suggestive of
the maxim that ' Might gives Right.'

The wind had now gone down, and there was
a pleasant light breeze, with a calm sea. The
scene was very animated; boats of all sorts and
sizes scattered about in every direction, steamers, steam launches, and row-boats, all passing
round and about the fleet; parties going on
board, and parties leaving the ship, with beautiful yachts of every rig, their snow-white sails
lighting up the scene as far as the eye could
reach.

It was now getting late, so we stood straight
across for Ryde, which we were not long in reach-

ing. A perfect fleet of yachts lay at anchor off the pier, and steamers from every part were busily disgorging their passengers, whilst the escaping steam kept up a continued hiss and roar. We soon brought up to the westward of the pier, and a boat came off to us which conveyed us ashore. We proceeded in due course to the Kent Hotel, where we were fortunate enough to procure rooms and a dinner.

The greater part of this evening I spent in finding a sailor to go with us on the morrow to our destination at Christchurch. Since I had been there some years back, the bar at the entrance of the harbour has shifted considerably, and but few of the Solent men knew anything of the place; in fact, they all look upon that coast with dread, it being a lee shore.

The town was crowded to repletion in consequence of the coming review, and the taps, the favourite resorts of the sailors, were in the most uproarious state. I had great difficulty in getting hold of anyone who knew the coast, and when I succeeded, the men preferred to obtain their fancy prices at Ryde to going on a cruize, others were so disgracefully inebriated as to be completely unable to talk sense. At last I got hold of a man who, though thoroughly intoxicated, was just able to make himself intelligible, and I thought perhaps by the morning he might sober down and answer our purpose. He was accordingly engaged and ordered to be on the pier at 8 A.M. next day.

The evening, sad to say, looked anything but promising. The wind had not changed, but a thick wet mist had set in, and we retired for the night, not without the gravest misgivings. At six next morning, I popped my head out of window, and sad to say, our worst anticipations were realised. It was a down-pour, a dead calm, and the wind south-west. Our only solace was that we should have the tide with us, which had not yet begun to ebb. It was quite clear that we should not now be able to get to Christchurch that night, but if we could reach Lymington we might proceed by train, leaving our boat within easy reach of home.

We found the skipper waiting for us at the entrance of the pier, and were soon again on board, but not a breath of air was to be felt, and the bergees hung from the mastheads of the various yachts anchored in the roads in the most melancholy manner. We paddled and drifted along with the tide, listening to the skipper, who was busy spinning yarns about himself and his belongings. He was a rough

diamond, and his language was not of the most
refined style. Amongst other tales, he told
us of an amusing 'sell' played upon him by his
mother, who had been in the habit of finding
fault with him for stealing her lucifer matches
to light his pipe. She had had resort to
every artifice in her power to protect them ;
she had hid them away, but he had always
managed to find them again, and she was in
despair. One fine morning, when he was about
to start on a long cruize, he discovered, to his
great delight, a new box full of matches, half of
which he clapped into his pockets, saying to
himself meanwhile : 'See here, mother's forgot to
hide her matches this morning, I take it she'll
miss a few when she comes to light the fire.' Off
he sets in great glee, and when, some distance
from land, he bethinks himself a pipe would be
comforting, having loaded his clay, with a
chuckle he produces the matches in question,
and to use his own words, ' I goes scrape, scrape,
scrape, one after t'other, but it wern't no good,
the tarnation things wouldn't light, so I knows
it wer a trick of mother's, and when I gets home
that night, mind-ee not having had a pipe all
day, I finds they'll strike fast eno' on mother's
box, but nohow elsèwhere, and I'm blest if them
there wern't a queer kind of match.'

The weather now began to thicken to windward, and a strong breeze worked up from the westward, against which we had to beat with the aid of the tide; it was not long before the glassy surface of the sea wore a stormy aspect, and there seemed every prospect of dirty weather setting in.   The wind and tide being contrary, a nasty sea rose, through which we rounded the Castle point at Cowes, and began to think it would be prudent to bring up there.   But as time was our object, we determined to hold on as long as we could, for hitherto we had got along famously. The wind, after leaving Cowes, moderated a little, and the sea in duty bound followed suit, the rain ceased, and we actually had a glimpse of the sun. These favourable circumstances tended greatly to encourage us, and the little ship ploughed along manfully through the waves.   As I have before narrated, we were complete novices in the art of working these Una-rigged boats, and the sailors we took on board as pilots were no wiser than ourselves; the result was that our reef tackle was all out of order, and we were forced to hold on under our full sail.

Thus we continued on our way, making the best use we could of the ebb tide. The tides in the Solent are most puzzling, and it is very necessary to engage a local man as pilot, unless great experience has been already acquired. The eddy tides, if artfully taken advantage of, are of the greatest assistance, as is proved every year at the regattas.

We continued to beat along, under the shore of the Isle of Wight, for a short distance further, when we made a board across to the northern shore, in order to get the ebb tide out of the Southampton water.

At about 3 P.M. we were nearing Lymington creek, and the weather had by this time become very stormy, the larger yachts had taken the precaution to shorten sail, but alas, we could not do so, and were obliged to hold on, all sail standing. The tide had now turned against us, and in order to enter the river, we were obliged to round a point known as ' Jack in the Basket,' beating against wind and tide. A nasty chopping sea had risen, which broke over and into us without mercy, obliging us to keep constantly baling out, and everytime we 'went about,' we had to shift the luggage, &c. to windward. In process of time we got round the point, and ran up the river at a great rate, the skipper steering by means of the main sheet as much as with the tiller, and at about four o'clock we dropped anchor in Lymington harbour.

The skipper, as before said, was a crusty sort of fellow, and he quarrelled with everyone who offered to lend us assistance or give us any information. One young sailor came up to me, and in passing some remarks about the 'Caprice,' pointed out another larger vessel which had originally been built as a Una boat, but a small bowsprit or 'bumpkin' had since been added to enable her to carry a jib. In alluding to her, he remarked, 'That's a nice Una boat, Sir.' Upon which our skipper turned upon him without mercy, and the following dialogue took place. 'You call that a Una boat, do you, perhaps you'll call yourself a seaman next.' 'Yes,' says the lad, 'I calls her a Una boat.' 'How can she be a Una boat, with two sails, you stupid fellow,' answers the skipper. 'Anyway she was built for one,' rejoined the youngster. 'D'ye call that the same thing,' says the skipper, 'I was built for a gentleman, but I aint one.'

The weather had by this time worked itself up to a gale, and craft of all rig came staggering into harbour under close-reefed canvas. This put an end to our further attempt to get to Christchurch. Alas! if the fine weather had but held on a few hours longer; still we had accomplished what we undertook, namely, the voyage from Weybridge to the Solent by canal and sea, and we were now compelled to bid adieu for the present to our little ship, whilst we took the train from Lymington to Christchurch.

At this point I think I ought to thank my readers for their perseverance in perusing this little tale. I only trust it may have proved amusing to some, I am sure it is suggestive of enterprise to those who are fond of sailing, and to those who possess a small sailing boat, and, having a few weeks' holiday from their daily work in London, may like to run down to the sea beyond the immediate precincts of London and the Thames, without much expenditure of either time or money.

CHAPTER VII.

ON THE UNA RIG, AND THE MANAGEMENT OF THE UNA BOAT—
ITS GREAT ADVANTAGES AS COMPARED WITH THE FORE-AND-
AFT RIG—VARIOUS SUGGESTIONS AND RECEIPTS FOR FITTING
OUT—AIR-TIGHT COMPARTMENTS—EXPERIMENTS TO TEST THEIR
EFFICACY—DUCK SHOOTING AT SEA IN THE UNA BOAT.

BEFORE bringing this little work to a close,
perhaps it would be well that I should make
some allusions to the capabilities of the Una
rig. Before I originally started a boat of this
kind, I had seen a good deal of sailing in yachts
of all sorts and sizes, and yachting has been,
and I hope always may be my hobby, but
l'homme propose et Dieu dispose, and my duty
called me to spend my existence within daily
reach of London, so I fixed my abode on the
banks of the Thames.

I soon found a fore-and-aft rigged boat was
of no use for river sailing. I could not get her
to beat to windward against the stream, and in
'going about' I was always obliged to help her
round with an oar, the greater part of the time
her nose being fast jammed in the mud banks.

The Una rig, on the contrary, is in my opinion exactly adapted for a river, for these boats will 'come round' like a top the instant the helm is put down. Of course there are exceptional cases; for instance, if a strong current is running against her, and there is not wind sufficient to get good way on, she will in all probability require a little help, but I may safely say that taking them all in all, there is nothing to come near them on lake or river—they sail closer to the wind than any others; the simplicity of the rig enables one 'hand' to manage them with ease (provided always that he knows what he is about), and the rapidity with which they answer their helm is surprising, whilst the smallest breath of wind is sufficient to propel them.

I was at first cautioned against Una boats, for I was told that they had an unpleasant tendency to turn upside down. This may be, I am happy to say, completely averted by means of having them built after the fashion of a lifeboat, with air-tight compartments; this cost me in my little boat an additional 10*l*., but query, Is not one's life worth 10*l*.? In my allusions to sea sailing, I shall have an opportunity of pointing out the great advantages of these air-tight compartments.

The 'Caprice' was built by Corke of Cowes,

and he, I believe, is the only man who builds
them with air-tight sides.   She measures 16 feet
in length from stem to stern, six feet beam, and
a foot and a half in depth ; she draws, with her
sliding-keel up, about eight inches, her deck
being eight inches above water, and is astonish-
ingly stiff, in fact I have never seen her in the
strongest breeze attempt to capsize ; the builder
informed me that he would guarantee her
against that, but he could not warrant her not
to fill.   Here he was right, for being so low in
the water, if a sudden squall heels her over in a
sea, or even in smooth water, she will take in a
considerable quantity, so that I have always
made it a rule never to go out without a good
serviceable baler.

When the boat was first sent to me, I found
some difficulty in fitting her out.   The sail in
this style of rig is laced to a long boom, which
projects nearly four feet over the stern.   The
boom is made very light and pliant, so much so
that at sea in a strong breeze, running before
the wind, the sail takes the shape of a bag, and
the boom at times bends to that degree, that
one almost fears it will snap.   I had some
thoughts of either having a heavier one, or the
present one weighted with lead, but on the
whole perhaps she is safer as she is, for in case
of a gibe, the lighter the boom the better.

For Thames sailing, we found her mast too long to pass under the bridges, even where the river was low in the middle of summer; we therefore rigged out a shorter one, 14 feet long, which we always use for river sailing, but, unfortunately, there is not length of mast sufficient to enable us to set up the whole sail; we are therefore always obliged to work her with one reef down; and it is amusing to hear the absurd remarks of the ignoramuses on the river, mocking at us for sailing in a light wind, almost becalmed, with a reef down, whereas, if they understood anything about sailing, they would at once see the cause.

The main and peak halliards in a Una boat are one and the same rope. In hoisting the sail, the end of the main halliards is made fast to the gaff about a foot or so from the point, this varies according to the set of the sail, and experience will decide its exact position. It is merely made fast by a double hitch, the rope then passes through the sheeve in a double block hooked at the mast-head, then through a single block near the jaws of the gaff, and up again mast high through the second sheeve of the double block, the end passing under a sheeve fastened to the deck before the mast, and belaying to a cleat inside the boat.

The topping lift is a very important rope. The boat, when sent to me originally, was not fitted with one, but I soon found that it was quite indispensable. The sail is so large that in reefing, the boom must be topped up, or when the sail is lowered, it will lower away into the water, and then it would not be long before the boat became thoroughly unmanageable. Again, it is most useful as a substitute for the main-tack, which does not exist in these boats, the sail being laced to the boom, and it is always called into play when the sail is furled, so that in ordering a Una boat great stress should be laid on her being fitted with a topping lift. This may be easily added in the following manner. Make fast one end of a rope to the end of the boom, pass it through a hole drilled in the mast-head, then through a sheeve on the deck similar to the one through which the main halliards work, one on each side of the mast; but mind, if these sheeves are made of iron, they must be galvanized, as everything of iron on board should be.

Next comes the most important of all points, that of reefing. When the boat reaches the purchaser, he will find that the end of the boom is so far away over the stern that he is unable to reach the first reef-thimble in order to pass his reef-earing through it; he should, therefore,. before he starts on his cruize, always see that he has one, if not two of his earings in good working order, the third may be worked inside the boat without difficulty. The way reefing is managed in a Una boat is thus :—two long and flat strips of wood are found to be securely screwed one on each side of the boom, just astern of the rudder. In each of these are drilled three holes large enough for the three reef-earings to work through with ease; they are exactly opposite each other, so that there are three pairs of holes about a foot apart. If the earings should not work easily through them, a red hot poker will burn away the wood and make a slanting smooth inclination towards the boat, which enables the reef to be hauled in easily, especially after a little grease has been applied. Now for the process of reefing itself: first take the earing, make a secure knot at one end, pass the other end from under one of the holes, draw it up taut, then pass it through the thimble on the sail, then through the opposite hole, haul away into the boat and make fast to the boom ; the remaining reefs are taken in the same way, only, for convenience sake, let the knot of the second reef-earing be under the opposite side of the boom to the first, and the third opposite to the second, which in a hurry may prevent confusion; by this means the sail will be hauled down flat on the boom, and may be reefed very quickly.

A word or two relative to the working of the main-sheet, and we shall have said all that is necessary about her running rigging—these boats have no standing rigging whatever. Two galvanised screws, with eyes, are let into the deck at the stern, one at each corner; and in a line with them on the boom, a small single block is fastened, and another small block is hooked to the port eye. The main-sheet is made fast to the starboard eye, then passes through the block on the boom, then through the block in the port eye, and belays to the cleat in the stern. This plan is better than a 'horse,' and works with the greatest facility and safety.

Now let us turn our attention to sea sailing. The 'Caprice,' as before said, was built essentially for smooth water; in fact, these boats, of whatever size, work better in calm weather. They are of all sizes, and in America are to be found of 50 tons and upwards; but I have been told that a boat of 10 tons of the Una rig is most serviceable. There is no doubt whatever they sail much nearer the wind in a smooth sea than any ordinary cutter rig, but in beating to windward in rough weather, they are very wet, and I find that my little boat is rather inclined to carry a lee helm in a chopping sea. I have rectified this in some measure by adding another hundredweight of ballast in the bows, which tends to steady her; besides which there are 160 lbs. of ballast in two rows, 80 lbs. on each side of the sliding keel.

Another most important point must be attended to if these boats are to be used for sea purposes, that is, to have their decks perfectly water-tight. The day we put into Lymington, we found this out to our cost, for the waves that washed over us penetrated through the seams on the deck, and poured in at the foot of the mast. This defect has since been remedied in the following manner :—viz., by covering the deck from stem to stern with stretched canvas, over which two good coats of paint have been added, and round the foot of the mast a kind of canvas bag has been nailed to the deck, which draws to and ties tight round the mast, about a foot above. This has exactly the desired effect.

The bulwarks are certainly not high enough for sea sailing, being only four inches in height; consequently, in bad weather, it often happens that we take in a very considerable quantity of water, and it is at these critical times that a good-sized baler is wanted. A boat twice the size would be safer and better adapted to sea sailing; but it has been suggested to me that she might be raised a plank higher out of the water, the deck being taken off and replaced, and bulwarks a foot higher substituted for the present ones. These should, I think, slant outwards in order to prevent the sea chopping into the boat; for when made upright, the waves, washing over the deck, dash against them, and bound up into the well. Such alterations would, however, spoil her outward appearance, and after all, she was originally built, and is more especially required, for river sailing, for which purpose no boat could be more perfectly adapted; and when dressed out with her white sail and bright flag, in her holiday attire, she looks exceedingly graceful and pretty.

One day, having nothing to do, and it blowing half a gale of wind, with violent squalls at intervals, I thought I could not do better than thoroughly test the efficiency of the air-tight compartments, so having procured a stout hand to help, we proceeded on board, and commenced operations by taking down two reefs; we then cleared everything out of her we could spare— mop, spars, ropes, &c. &c., pulled out the plug at the bottom, and set forth on our cruise over the mud banks in the harbour, it being high tide at the time. Before long the water inside became flush with that outside, and she ceased filling further; all this time she sailed first rate, being completely manageable, and the more she took in, the stiffer she became. We then began to fill her still fuller with a bucket, until she completely settled down below the water-line. She sailed as well as ever, and answered her helm perfectly. In fact it became now very difficult for us to keep inside at all, as the tendency was for her to sail away from under *us*, whilst we floated out of *her*; this proving that if the worst came to the worst, she would not sink, but we should be washed out in a sea, if not lashed to something on board. A terribly spiteful squall now struck us, which sent her over on her beam ends, bringing the sail almost into the water; this, of course, could not be permitted, or she would have *bonâ fide* capsized, so we were forced to luff her up, and she then righted at once. The wind and rain, meanwhile, were coming down in a perfect fury, completely blinding us, and the surface of the water was torn up into quite a sea; whilst we had great difficulty in both steering and keeping in her, the lee gunwale being altogether invisible under water. At this moment, a peal of thunder burst over our heads with ominous effect. We had to ride out this storm for some time drenched to the skin, for we had not thought it wise to wrap ourselves in water-proof clothes, for fear we might have to swim for it, in which case the less we had on the better. Several boats put out to our assistance, unable to comprehend our movements. But there is an end to all things; in time the storm calmed down a bit, and having thoroughly tested our gallant little ship with the most satisfactory results, we commenced to bucket out the water, and to make for our moorings.

The little 'Caprice' is a source of great amusement to us, there being very few days when the weather is too stormy to go out to sea, small as she is; at which times we have always great fun cruising about the harbour after coot, dabchicks, and at times higher game. In the summer we found her very use-ful for mackerel and whiting fishing, for we could run out in no time to the ledge of rocks off Hengisbury Head, about three miles distant, lower away the sail, and commence operations.

On this ledge the fishermen of Mudiford place their lobster and prawn pots, which, as most people know, have long lines attached to them, on which numbers of corks are strung, about a foot apart, these are marked in some particular way to distinguish one man's pots from another, and as they float on the top of the water, they indicate the position of the pots themselves. They proved a great nuisance to us, for they were continually getting hung up in the rudder, and one day we nearly came to grief in consequence.

We had been out for an hour or two's cruise off the ledge, when we were suddenly 'brought-up' by one of these lines getting jammed in the rudder, and anchoring us most effectually by the stern. As always happens when anything goes wrong in a boat, the wind at once began to rise, and the sea accordingly ; still, do what we would, we could not get free. Meanwhile the waves were washing in over the stern, and our position did not seem an enviable one ; a naval officer who was with us remarking, with rather a blue face, that we *must* be swamped. It at last occurred to us that we had better get the sail down, which we did, and after working away at the helm, we succeeded at last in extricating ourselves. We had not proceeded twenty yards before we were brought up a second time in like manner, but experience having taught us, we lost no time in lowering

the sail, which prevented the line from becoming so tightly jammed, and we got free
much sooner than before.

These mishaps, however, proved to us that
some remedy must be provided against a repe-
tition of such an occurrence, for in a rough
sea one might fare badly, if arrested on one's
course in so peremptory a manner. After consulting the fishermen, I found that the plan
they adopted was to have what they call a
'shoe' placed under the rudder and keel.
This 'shoe' consists of a thin piece of iron
about eight inches long, the width of the keel,
which is nailed to it, having four inches pro-
truding, on the top of which the rudder rests,
so that by this means nothing can get between
them. Since I have had this 'shoe' put to my
boat, I have sailed perpetually among the pot-
lines without let or hindrance.

There is another annoyance in sea sailing,
which it will be well to mention; namely, the
weeds, which in summer grow in such profusion,
and in an incredibly short space of time. On
our arrival at the sea we had our boat thoroughly fitted out, and two coats of paint laid
on outside and in, but a fortnight had not
elapsed before we had to beach her again, and
give her bottom a good scrubbing to clear her

from the weeds, in doing which we were forced
to scrape off all the paint we had so lately
put on. On enquiry I discovered that the
fishermen at Mudiford make a concoction of
half pitch and common varnish, with which
they anoint the bottoms of their boats; this
does not keep off the weeds, but they do not
grow so quickly, and when the boat is cleaned,
this stuff does not scrape off, but works into the
wood and preserves it from rotting. For sea
boats, Stockholm tar is very useful, but in fresh
water it is as useless as paint for protecting the
wood. There is, however, a liquid called me-
tallic paint, sold by Mr. William Day, of Gloster
Place, Salmon's Lane, E.C., London, which
answers the double purpose of preserving the
wood and preventing the weeds from growing.

Of one thing I am perfectly convinced,
that no boat is constructed which is better
adapted for wildfowl shooting than a Una. I
have had great sport off the coast, cruizing
about after birds, and my experience has proved
to me that there are but very few days when
it is worth while going in quest of birds at
sea, that the weather would be unfit for a
small Una boat; for if the sea be rough, birds
are wild and restless, and would not let any
boat get near them—added to which, who can

H

see birds any distance in a lumpy sea? or who can shoot from a boat rolling about? to say nothing of picking up the wounded, every one of which would get away. In moderate weather a Una boat sails so fast that she is down upon the birds before they are aware of her presence, she cuts through the water so quietly, without the plunging and lobbing gait of a heavy sea-going boat, that she steals up to them quite unawares. Then again, in chasing cripples, there is nothing to equal these boats, for they 'come about' at once, and are off again before a fore-and-aft boat can get round. In chasing grebe and divers of all kinds, they are invaluable, they will work with the smallest amount of wind, and when any other boat is almost becalmed, a Una will go ahead with ease.

We have a fore-and-aft boat for bad weather, and the Una for fine weather, and up to the time at which I write, the preference, as far as regards wild-fowl shooting, is decidedly in favour of the latter, but for fishing, the fore-and-aft boat will work a trawl, whilst the Una will not, being too light.

Very often, in the 'Caprice,' I have been able to beat against the tide, sailing so close to the wind, and being so short a time 'in stays,' that I have accomplished what no ordinary boat would attempt, and where you must take advantage of everything in your power when wildfowl are near, this has proved of the greatest utility in enabling me to get the first start.

My boat being white, I have provided for myself and companions white linen jackets sufficiently large to slip on over any amount of warm clothing, which, with white woollen caps, enable us to get nearer the birds. Given a Una boat twice the size of mine, and a good double-duck gun No. 8 guage—it is a man's own fault if he does not see sport.

I hope that some of the foregoing hints may be of use. I have written them on the presumption that all who read this chapter are acquainted with the ordinary nautical terms. Should anyone not versed in these matters wish to get hold of a really useful practical work on sailing, I would recommend very strongly Mr. Folkard's little book, called the ' Sailing Boat,' published by Messrs. Longman and Co.

It now only remains for me to bid my readers farewell, and if any of them should be possessed of a Una boat, I cannot do better than express the hope that they may have as much fun with theirs as I have with mine.

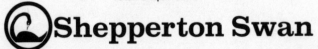